Air Fryer Oven Toaster

Mastering Cookbook

Making the Most of Your Air

Fryer with 50 Recipes That Will

Delight Your Family and

Friends

By

Ronda William

Respective authors own all copyrights not held by the publisher.

The information herein is offered for informational purposes solely and is universal as so. The presentation of the information is without a contract or any type of guarantee assurance.

The trademarks that are used are without any consent, and the publication of the trademark is without permission or backing by the trademark owner. All trademarks and brands within this book are for clarifying purposes only and are owned by the owners themselves, not affiliated with this document.

Table of Contents

Conclusion

Introduction

Air fryers have become very popular appliances, and since they appeared, they have given much to talk about their uses and benefits, one of the best known: frying without using oil or with a very little amount of oil. Air fryers are appliances that use hot air to fry food in a healthy way. Among the many benefits of these appliances is that they are easy to use and clean, do not emit frying odors and reduce the intake of fat and cholesterol from foods fried in oils.

However, it should not be forgotten that there is a toxic compound called acrylamide, which is believed to be carcinogenic and appears in certain foods when they are fried when heated to temperatures above 120°C and in contact with the oil, so it is recommended to eat raw, natural and whole foods because it is almost always the healthiest option. However, with an air fryer, without oil, you can cook foods with very little fat content and with the texture and flavor similar to fried foods, without the inconvenience that frying brings to health.

The key is to maintain a healthy and balanced diet without neglecting to eat in a delicious and nutritious way, preserving food juices and nutrients. Of course, we cannot leave aside other options for cooking food, since eating everything fried can obviously cause health problems in the long run.

Chapter 1: Breakfast and

Brunch Recipes

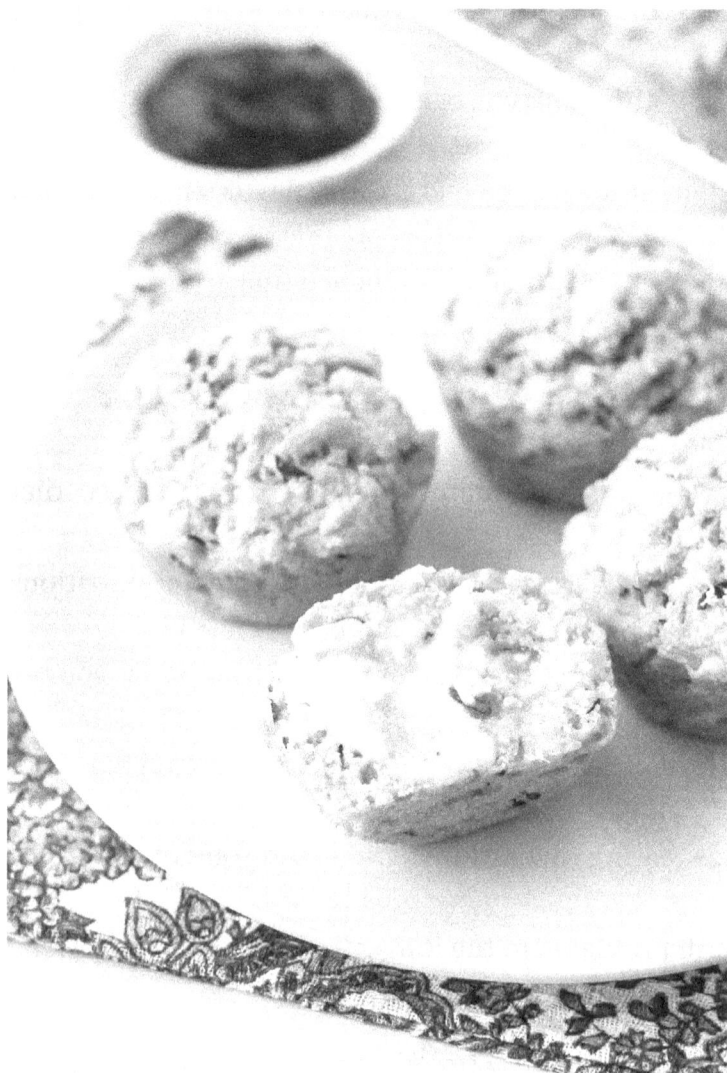

1. Cornbread Zucchini Muffins

(Ready in about 30 minutes | **Serving:** 6 | **Difficulty**: Easy)

Per serving: **Kcal** 157, **Fat**: 6 g, **Net Carbs**: 23 g, **Protein**: 5 g

Ingredients:

- 1 cup shredded zucchini squash

- ½ cup cornmeal yellow

- ½ cup whole-wheat white flour

- 1 tablespoon granulated sugar

- 1 teaspoon baking powder

- 1/8 teaspoon baking soda

- ½ teaspoon salt

- 1 beaten egg

- ¼ cup whole milk

- ¼ cup low-fat plain yogurt

- 2 tablespoons melted unsalted butter, cooled

- ¼ cup drained canned corn

- Oil

Instructions:

1. Preheat the air fryer to 350°F. Oil a muffin pan gently and cut ends of zucchini. Use a box grate to grate zucchini. Add zucchini with all the ingredients in a bowl and mix thoroughly. Add batter to cups of muffin pan evenly. Cook for around 15 minutes.

2. Broiled Mango

(Ready in about 10 minutes | **Serving:** 2 | **Difficulty**: Easy)

Per serving: **Kcal** 162, **Fat**: 1 g, **Net Carbs**: 33 g, **Protein**: 10 g

Ingredients:

- 1 large ripe mango

- ½ teaspoon sugar

- 1/8–¼ teaspoon chili powder

- A pinch of sea salt

Optional Toppings:

- Coconut Flakes Cooked

- Granola

- Cooked Nuts

Instructions:

1. Slice each side of the mango carefully and score the flesh with a paring knife. Sprinkle with chili powder, sugar, and salt. Place the mango on a pan and cook for around 5 minutes.

3. Mini Eggless Bread

(Ready in about 40 minutes | **Serving:** 1 | **Difficulty**: Easy)

Per serving: **Kcal** 138, **Fat**: 6 g, **Net Carbs**: 21 g, **Protein**: 2 g

Ingredients:

Dry:

- ½ cup whole-wheat white flour

- ¼ teaspoon baking powder

- ¼ teaspoon baking soda

- ¼ teaspoon cinnamon

- 1/8 teaspoon table salt

Wet:

- ½ cup banana mashed

- 1 tablespoon cane sugar organic

- 2 tablespoon brown sugar packed

- 2 tablespoon canola oil

- ½ teaspoon lemon juice

- ¼ teaspoon vanilla extract pure

Instructions:

1. Preheat the air fryer to 350°F. Oil a pan gently and mix dry ingredients in a bowl. Use another bowl to mix the wet ingredients and combine both mixtures. Pour mixture into the pan and cook for around 25 minutes.

4. Frittata

(Ready in about 50 minutes | **Serving: 2** | **Difficulty**: Moderate)

Per serving: **Kcal** 265, **Fat**: 19 g, **Net Carbs**: 9 g, **Protein**: 17 g

Ingredients:

- 2 teaspoons divided grapeseed oil
- ½ cup thinly sliced brussels sprouts

- 1/2 cup chopped broccoli florets

- 2–3 chopped cremini mushrooms

- 1 thinly sliced shallot

- 1/4 teaspoon dried oregano

- Salt and pepper, as per taste

- 2 tablespoons feta cheese crumbled

- ½ chopped red pepper, roasted

- 4 eggs

- 2 tablespoons half-and-half

- 1 tablespoon finely chopped fresh herbs, thyme, or parsley

- ¼ teaspoon sea salt

- 1/8 teaspoon black pepper

Instructions:

1. Preheat the air fryer to 400°F. Oil a pan gently. Add vegetables to the pan and drizzle with the rest of the oil. Season using pepper and salt. Mix vegetables to coat. Cook the mixture for around 15 minutes. Mix eggs, salt, half-and-half, herbs, and pepper in a bowl. Take the pan out of the oven and sprinkle red pepper and feta over. Pour bowl mixture on top and cook for another 20 minutes.

Chapter 2: Fish and

Seafood Recipes

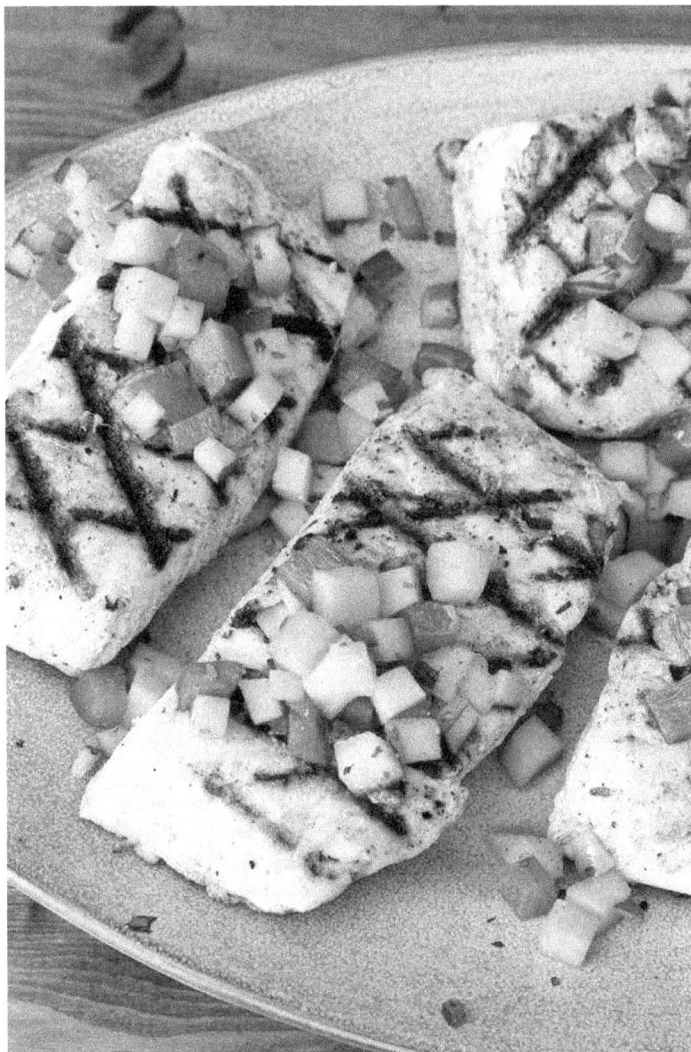

5. Crispy Shrimp

(Ready in about 15 minutes | **Serving:** 4 | **Difficulty**:

Easy)

Per serving: **Kcal:** 140, **Fat**: 4 g, **Net Carbs**: 3 g,

Protein: 4 g

Ingredients:

- 12 peeled and deveined big shrimp

- 2 egg whites

- 1 cup shredded coconut

- 1 cup panko crumbs

- 1 cup white flour

- Salt

- Black pepper

Instructions:

1. Mix coconut and panko in a bowl. Add pepper, salt, and flour in another bowl and whisk whites of eggs in a separate bowl. Dip shrimp using flour, then whites and coconut at the end. Place them in the basket of the fryer and broil for around 10 minutes at 350°F.

6. Flavored Salmon

(Ready in about 1 hour 8 minutes | **Serving:** 2 | **Difficulty**: Hard)

Per serving: **Kcal:** 300, **Fat**: 12 g, **Net Carbs**: 23 g, **Protein**: 20 g

Ingredients:

- 2 salmon fillets

- 2 tablespoons lemon juice

- Salt

- Black pepper

- ½ teaspoon garlic powder

- 1/3 cup water

- 1/3 cup soy sauce

- 3 chopped scallions

- 1/3 cup brown sugar

- 2 tablespoons olive oil

Instructions:

1. Add all the ingredients except scallions in a bowl and toss to combine thoroughly. Place in the fridge for around an hour and place in a basket

of the fryer. Broil for around 8 minutes at 360°F. Sprinkle scallions and enjoy.

7. Delicious Catfish

(Ready in about 30 minutes | **Serving:** 4 | **Difficulty**: Easy)

Per serving: **Kcal:** 253, **Fat**: 6 g, **Net Carbs**: 26 g, **Protein**: 22 g

Ingredients:

- 4 fillets catfish

- Salt

- Black pepper

- A pinch of sweet paprika

- 1 tablespoon chopped parsley

- 1 tablespoon lemon juice

- 1 tablespoon olive oil

Instructions:

1. Season catfish with seasonings and rub oil over it. Place in the basket of the fryer and broil for around 10 minutes at 400°F. Drizzle using lemon juice and enjoy.

8. Cajun Shrimp

(Ready in about 15 minutes | **Serving:** 2 | **Difficulty**: Easy)

Per serving: **Kcal:** 162, **Fat:** 6 g, **Net Carbs**: 8 g, **Protein**: 14 g

Ingredients:

- 20 tiger shrimp, deveined and peeled

- Salt

- Black pepper

- ½ teaspoon seasoning old bay

- 1 tablespoon olive oil

- ¼ teaspoon smoked paprika

Instructions:

1. Add all the ingredients in a bowl with shrimp and mix to coat thoroughly. Place shrimp in the basket of the fryer and broil for around 5 minutes at 390°F.

Chapter 3: Snacks,

Appetizers, and Sides

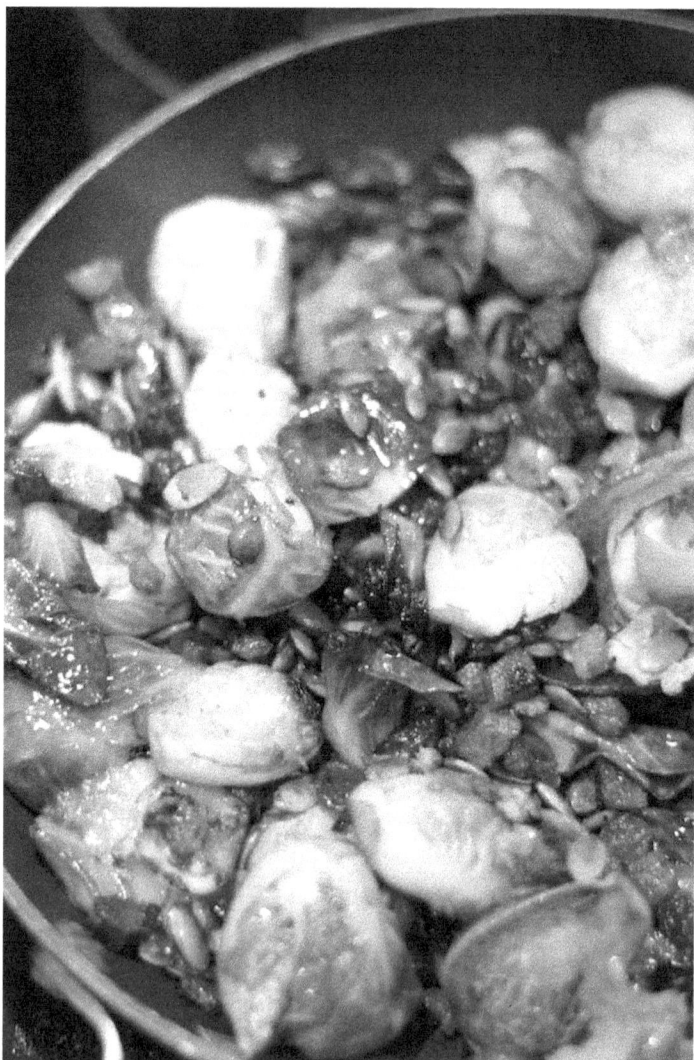

9. Brussels Sprouts & Pancetta

(Ready in about 25 minutes | **Serving**: 4 | **Difficulty**: Easy)

Per serving: **Kcal:** 108, **Fat**: 6 g, **Net Carbs**: 11 g, **Protein**: 5 g

Ingredients:

- 1 lb. trimmed Brussels sprouts, halved

- 1 thinly sliced shallot

- 1 oz. diced pancetta

- 1 tablespoon olive oil

- 1/8 teaspoon kosher salt

- 1/8 teaspoon black pepper, freshly ground

- 2 teaspoons wine vinegar

Instructions:

1. Line a pan with aluminum foil and add all ingredients except vinegar in the pan. Toss to coat evenly. Place pan in the fryer and cook for around 15 minutes at 400°F. They will become tender and crispy. Transfer them to a bowl and mix with vinegar.

10. Beet Chips Fresh Dill

(Ready in about 15 minutes | **Serving**: 2 | **Difficulty**: Easy)

Per serving: **Kcal**: 51, **Fat**: 2 g, **Net Carbs**: 7 g, **Protein**: 1 g

Ingredients:

- 5 oz. beet

- Cooking spray

- ¼ teaspoon kosher salt

- 1 tablespoon chopped fresh dill

- ½ teaspoon wine vinegar

Instructions:

1. Cut beet into fine slices and add to the basket of the fryer. Spray the oil over and sprinkle salt. Place the basket inside the fryer and cook for around 5 minutes at 400°F. The edges will become crispy and turn brown. Transfer to a bowl and sprinkle with vinegar and dill.

11. Shrimp Diablo

(Ready in about 70 minutes | **Serving**: 5 | **Difficulty**: Hard)

Per serving: **Kcal:** 283, **Fat**: 20 g, **Net Carbs**: 14 g, **Protein**: 14 g

Ingredients:

- ¼ cup EVOO

- 2 smashed garlic cloves

- 1½ teaspoon red pepper, crushed

- 28 oz. roughly chopped plum tomatoes, whole

- 2¼ teaspoon kosher salt

- 1 lb. large shrimp, cleaned, peeled, and rinsed

- ¼ cup rice flour white

- Sauce to serve

Instructions:

1. Add garlic, red pepper, and olive oil to a pan and simmer for around 15 minutes. Add tomatoes and simmer for around 30 more minutes. Add 3/4 teaspoon of salt. Sprinkle shrimp with the rest of the salt and coat using rice flour. Place basket on the pan and add shrimp and spray using olive oil. Cook for around 10 minutes at 375°F. Serve with sauce, and enjoy.

12. Gruyère, Spinach and Artichoke Dip

(Ready in about 35 minutes | **Serving**: 2 | **Difficulty**: Easy)

Per serving: **Kcal:** 99, **Fat:** 7 g, **Net Carbs**: 5 g, **Protein**: 5 g

Ingredients:

- Olive oil to grease

- 12 oz. cream cheese, 1" pieces

- 2 oz. finely grated Gruyère cheese

- 1 oz. finely grated Parmesan cheese

- 1 finely chopped garlic clove

- ½ small finely chopped shallot

- 8 oz. thawed and well-drained spinach

- 15 oz. drained artichoke hearts, quartered

- 2 tablespoon heavy cream

- ½ teaspoon red pepper, crushed

Instructions:

1. Coat a pan with oil. Add cream cheese to a bowl and mix with a hand mixer. Add the rest of the ingredients and combine thoroughly. Pour mixture on the pan and cook for around 20 minutes at 350°F.

13. Spring Rolls & Dipping Sauce

(Ready in about 30 minutes | **Serving**: 8 | **Difficulty**: Easy)

Per serving: **Kcal:** 14, **Fat**: 0 g, **Net Carbs**: 3 g, **Protein**: 0 g

Ingredients:

Dipping Sauce:

- 1 red chili, sliced into 1" slices

- 1 smashed garlic clove

- 1 tablespoon unsweetened rice wine vinegar

- 1 cup water

- 1/3 cup sugar granulates

- 1 tablespoon + 1 teaspoon cornstarch, in 1 tablespoon water

- ¼ teaspoon kosher salt

Spring Rolls:

- 6 cabbage leaves green, thinly sliced

- 3 julienned medium carrots

- 1" piece julienned fresh ginger

- 3 thinly sliced green onions

- ½ green chile, small

- 1/3 cup thinly sliced basil leaves, fresh

- ½ cup chopped cilantro leaves, fresh

- 2 tablespoon vegetable oil

- 1 tablespoon fish sauce

- ½ juiced lime

- ½ teaspoon kosher salt

- ½ block tofu, extra-firm sliced in 28 thick julienne strips

- 28 wrappers egg roll

Instructions:

1. Add garlic and chili slices in a pot and warm until it is fragrant. Take off the flame and

vinegar. Place on the flame to reduce vinegar. Add sugar and water and boil the mixture. Add a mixture of cornstarch and boil for around one minute. Take off the flame and add salt. Blend in a blender until garlic and chili slices are pureed.

2. Add filling ingredients in a bowl except for tofu and mix. Put a basket of the fryer on the pan. Place one tofu piece in the middle of each wrapper and add 1 tablespoon of filling. Fold bottom over filling in the upward direction. Coat water at the edges and place it in the basket. Drizzle rolls with oil and does with the rest of the wrappers as well. Cook for around 10 minutes at 400°F.

14. French Fries

(Ready in about 25 minutes | **Serving**: 3 | **Difficulty**:

Easy)

Per serving: **Kcal:** 138, **Fat**: 2 g, **Net Carbs**: 27 g,

Protein: 4 g

Ingredients:

- 1 lb. russet potatoes

- Cooking spray

- 1 teaspoon kosher salt

Instructions:

1. Slice potatoes into pieces of 1/4 inch. Place a

   basket of the fryer on the pan and add potatoes.

Spray oil and add salt. Cook for around 15 minutes at 400°F.

15. Ginger and Pork Wontons

(Ready in about 25 minutes | **Serving**: 48 | **Difficulty**: Easy)

Per serving: **Kcal:** 141, **Fat:** 6 g, **Net Carbs**: 14 g, **Protein**: 8 g

Ingredients:

- ¾ lb. minced pork

- 3" piece chopped ginger

- 1 large chopped green onion

- 1 tablespoon freshly chopped cilantro leaves

- 1 tablespoon reduced-sodium soy sauce

- 2 teaspoons sesame oil

- ½ teaspoon rice vinegar

- Water and cornstarch for dumplings assembly

- 48 wonton-wrappers

- A drizzle of vegetable oil

Instructions:

1. Mix ginger, cilantro, pork, green onion, sesame oil, soy sauce, and vinegar in a bowl. Mix thoroughly. Add water to one bowl and cornstarch to another. Sprinkle cornstarch on the work surface and make rows of wonton wrappers. Add 1 teaspoon of filling in the middle of every wrapper. Brush edges with water and makes a triangle by folding in half. Do with the

rest of the wrappers and filling and toss with cornstarch. Place basket o fryer on pan and spray. Add half of the wontons in the basket and drizzle oil. Cook for around 10 minutes at 375°F. Repeat with the rest of the wontons.

16. Acorn Squash Roasted

(Ready in about 35 minutes | **Serving**: 4 | **Difficulty**: Easy)

Per serving: **Kcal:** 104, **Fat**: 1 g, **Net Carbs**: 24 g, **Protein**: 3 g

Ingredients:

- 1 teaspoon EVOO

- 1 acorn squash (in 12 wedges)

- ½ teaspoon kosher salt

- ¼ teaspoon black pepper, freshly ground

- ¼ teaspoon chili powder

Instructions:

1. Drizzle a pan with oil and add squash. Sprinkle pepper, salt, and chili powder. Place pan in the fryer and cook for around 25 minutes at 400°F. It will be soft and browned evenly.

17. Roasted Carrots, Fennel, and Parsnips

(Ready in about 40 minutes | **Serving**: 4 | **Difficulty**: Easy)

Per serving: **Kcal**: 170, **Fat**: 11 g, **Net Carbs**: 18 g,

Protein: 2 g

Ingredients:

- 2 trimmed fennel bulbs, quartered

- 3 carrots, medium (1" pieces)

- 1 parsnip, large (1" pieces)

- 1 smashed garlic clove

- 3 tablespoons EVOO

- ½ teaspoon kosher salt

- ¼ teaspoon black pepper

- A pinch of ground cinnamon

- 1 teaspoon thyme leaves, fresh

Instructions:

1. Add all the ingredients to a pan and mix. For a single layer of mixture and place the pan in the fryer. Cook for around 20 minutes at 400°F. The vegetables will turn tender, and the color will be slightly brown.

18. Chicken Dip

(Ready in about 35 minutes | **Serving:** 10 | **Difficulty**: Easy)

Per serving: **Kcal:** 240, **Fat**: 10 g, **Net Carbs**: 24 g, **Protein**: 12 g

Ingredients:

- 3 tablespoons melted butter
- 1 cup yogurt

- 12 oz. cream cheese

- 2 cups shredded chicken meat

- 2 teaspoons curry powder

- 4 chopped scallions

- 6 oz. Monterey jack grated cheese

- 1/3 cup raisins

- ¼ cup chopped cilantro

- ½ cup sliced almonds

- Salt

- Black pepper

- ½ cup chutney

Instructions:

1. In a dish, add cream cheese, yogurt and mix using your mixer. Add curry powder, scallions, chicken meat, raisins, cheese, cilantro, salt, and pepper and mix everything. Spread into the tray and put it in the fryer, sprinkle almonds on it, put it in the fryer, toast at 300°F for twenty minutes. Serve it in bowls along with some side servings.

19. Sweet Fries with Chipotle Mayonnaise

(Ready in about 30 minutes | **Serving**: 3 | **Difficulty**: Easy)

Per serving: **Kcal**: 101, **Fat**: 11 g, **Net Carbs**: 0 g, **Protein**: 0 g

Ingredients:

Chipotle Mayonnaise:

- ½ cup mayonnaise

- 1 finely chopped chipotle chile with adobo

- ¼ teaspoon lemon juice

Sweet Potato:

- 1 lb. sweet potatoes, ¼" thick, and 4" long

- olive oil

- ½ teaspoon kosher salt

Instructions:

1. Add lemon juice, chipotle, and mayonnaise in a food processor and puree. Pour into a bowl and refrigerate. Add a basket of the fryer to a pan and spray potatoes with oil. Sprinkle salt and mix. Make a single layer and cook for around 15 minutes at 400°F. They will become crispy and golden. Serve with sauce and enjoy.

Chapter 4: Beef Recipes

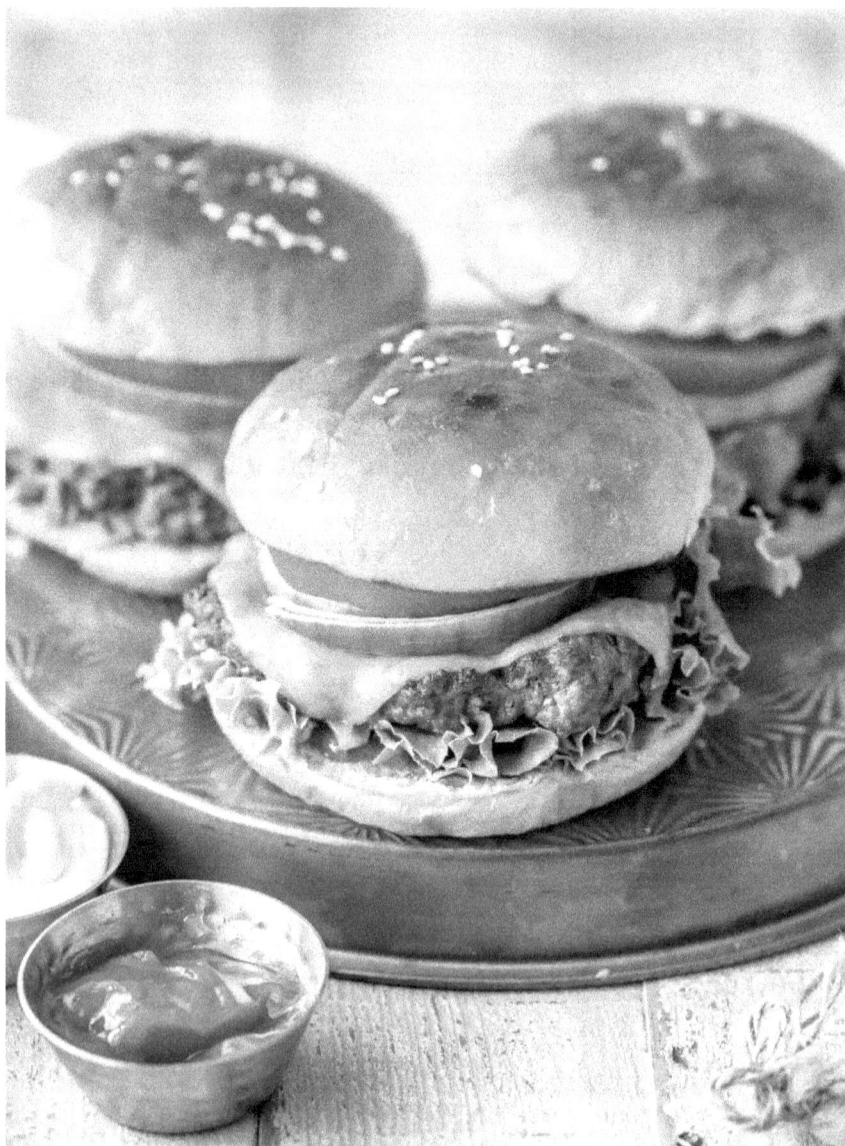

20. Hamburgers

(Ready in about 25 minutes | **Serving:** 4 | **Difficulty**:

Easy)

Per serving: **Kcal:** 528, **Fat:** 26 g, **Net Carbs**: 33 g,

Protein: 39 g

Ingredients:

- 1 ½ lb. ground beef

- 1 finely chopped small onion

- 1 egg

- ½ cup breadcrumbs

- ¼ cup bits of bacon

- Garlic salt as per taste

- 4 toasted and split hamburger buns

Instructions:

1. Preheat the air fryer to 360°F. Mix the beef, egg, onion, bacon bits, and breadcrumbs in a bowl. Use garlic salt to season. Make four balls of the mixture, and shape them into patties. Oil the basket gently and place patties inside. Broil each side for around 5 minutes.

21. Munroe Melt

(Ready in about 10 minutes | **Serving:** 1 | **Difficulty**:

Easy)

Per serving: **Kcal:** 835, **Fat**: 38 g, **Net Carbs**: 76 g,

Protein: 47 g

Ingredients:

- 1 crusty split sandwich roll

- 1 tablespoon prepared mayonnaise Dijon

  mustard mix

- 2 deli turkey slices

- 1 Swiss cheese slice

- 2 deli ham slices

- 1 tablespoon mayonnaise

- 2 deli beef roast slices

- 2 tomato slices

- 1 Muenster cheese slice

Instructions:

1. Preheat the air fryer to 360°F. Use aluminum foil to line a baking sheet. On the lined baking sheet, expand the sandwich roll. On one part of the roll, scatter the mayonnaise-mustard mixture and cover it with Swiss cheese, turkey, and ham. On the rest of the roll, spread 1 tablespoon mayonnaise and cover with the tomato slices, beef, and the Muenster cheese. Broil in the air fryer until the cheese melts.

22. Beef with Cabbage

(Ready in about 50 minutes | **Serving:** 6 | **Difficulty**: Easy)

Per serving: **Kcal:** 353, **Fat**: 16 g, **Net Carbs**: 20 g, **Protein**: 24 g

Ingredients:

- 2 and 1/2 pounds of beef brisket

- 1 cup beef stock

- 2 bay leaves

- 3 chopped garlic cloves

- 4 chopped carrots

- 1 diced cabbage head medium wedges

- Black pepper and salt

- 3 turnips, diced into quarters

Instructions:

1. Add stock and beef brisket in a pan and season beef using pepper and salt. Add the rest of the ingredients and toss. Place in the fryer and broil for around 40 minutes at 360°F.

23. Turkish Kebabs

(Ready in about 24 hours | **Serving:** 6 | **Difficulty**:

Hard)

Per serving: **Kcal:** 512, **Fat**: 34 g, **Net Carbs**: 36 g,

Protein: 16 g

Ingredients:

Marinade:

- 2 chopped large onions

- 2 crushed garlic cloves

- ½ cup olive oil

- 1 teaspoon dried oregano

- 2 tablespoon lemon juice

- 1 teaspoon black pepper

- 1 pinch of curry powder

- ½ teaspoon ground turmeric

- 1 teaspoon salt

- 1 lb. flank steak, beef thinly sliced

Sauce:

- 8 oz. sour cream

- 1 tablespoon lemon juice

- 2 tablespoon olive oil

- ½ teaspoon salt

- 1 tablespoon dill chopped

- 1 crushed garlic clove

- 6 rounds pita bread

- ½ teaspoon black pepper

Instructions:

1. In a bowl, add the sliced onions and smash until juice is created using the bottom side of the glass. Mix in 2 cloves of garlic (crushed), 1/2 cup of olive oil, curry powder, turmeric, 2 teaspoons of lemon juice, oregano, and 1 teaspoon each of black pepper and of salt. Mix well; apply the diced beef and mix. Wrap the bowl, then marinate overnight in the fridge. Mix the 2 tablespoons of olive oil, sour cream, 1 tablespoon of lemon juice, 1/2 teaspoon of the cinnamon, dill, 1/2 teaspoon of the black pepper, and 1 minced garlic clove. Mix well; wrap and place in the fridge overnight. Preheat the air fryer to 360°F. Take the beef out of the

marinade and dust off the excess onions. Place the slices, without overlapping, on a baking sheet and apply salt to taste. Broil each side for around 3 minutes. Divide the meat among the pita bread and drizzle using tzatziki sauce.

Chapter 5: Bakery and

Desserts

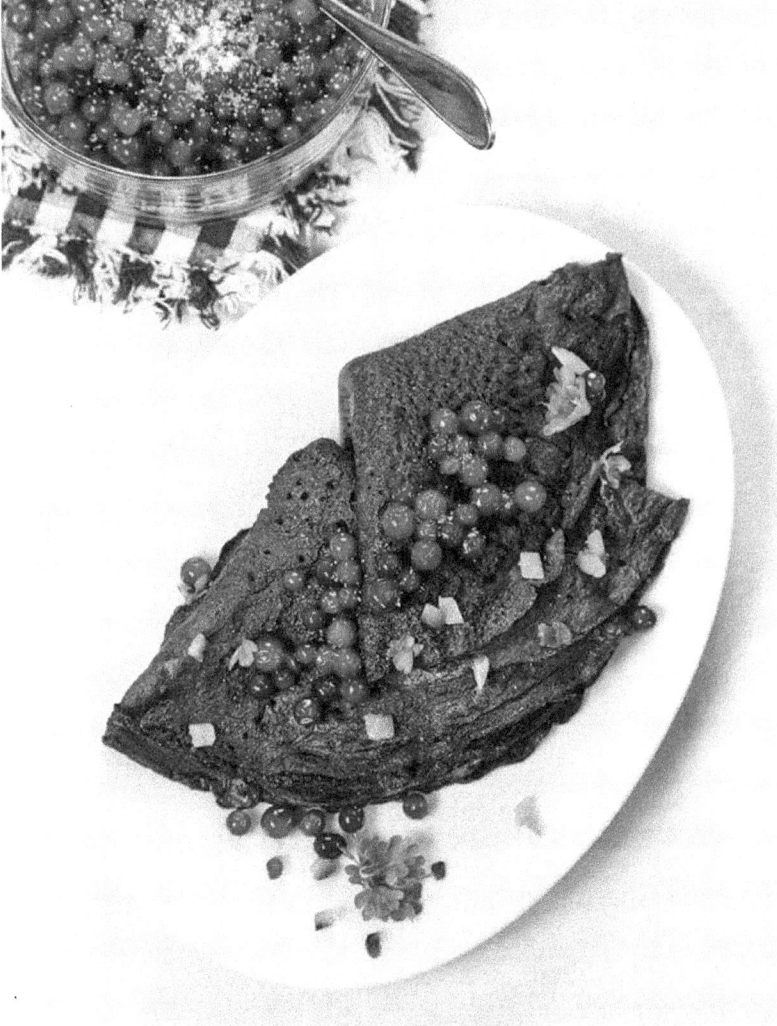

24. Flatbread Pizza

(Ready in about 28 minutes | **Serving:** 1 | **Difficulty**:

Easy)

Per serving: **Kcal**: 248, **Fat**: 9 g, **Net Carbs**: 35 g,

Protein: 10 g

Ingredients:

- 2 tablespoons flaked coconut unsweetened

- 1 naan whole-wheat flatbread

- ½ teaspoon coconut oil melted

- ¼ teaspoon cinnamon

- A pinch of sea salt, fine grain

- ¼ cup whole-milk ricotta cheese

- 2 teaspoons lemon curd prepared

- 8 oz. mixed berries, fresh

- Lemon zest, freshly grated

- Mint leaves fresh

Instructions:

1. Preheat fryer at 325°F. Cook coconuts in the pan for 3 to 6 minutes and set aside. Prepare the flatbread with coconut oil, cinnamon, and salt. Toast the flatbread for 7 to 8 minutes and cool. Mix ricotta with lemon curd. Put ricotta mixture, berries, coconut, lemon zest, and mint on flatbread and serve.

25. Coffee Parfaits

(Ready in about 10 minutes | **Serving:** 2 | **Difficulty**:

Easy)

Per serving: **Kcal**: 196, **Fat**: 7 g, **Net Carbs**: 23 g,

Protein: 11 g

Ingredients:

- ½ cup plain non-fat Greek yogurt

- 1/8 teaspoon instant espresso, finely ground

- ¼ teaspoon maple syrup, real

- 1/8 teaspoon vanilla extract, pure

- ½ cup almond granola, small batch

- ½ cup chopped and seeded cherries

Instructions:

1. Mix all the ingredients in a small bowl. Take two
    8 ounce jars, layer granola, cherries, and yogurt,
    and repeat the layers to make parfaits. Cool and
    serve.

26. Cookies

(Ready in about 27 minutes | **Serving:** 6 | **Difficulty**: Easy)

Per serving: **Kcal**: 104, **Fat**: 6 g, **Net Carbs**: 14 g, **Protein**: 2 g

Ingredients:

- 1 ½ tablespoon softened unsalted butter

- 3 tablespoon brown sugar

- 1 egg yolk, large, save white for later use

- ¼ teaspoon vanilla extract

- 2 tablespoon baking cocoa, unsweetened

- ¼ cup whole-wheat white flour

- ¼ teaspoon baking soda

- A pinch of sea salt

- 3 tablespoon divided chocolate chips

Instructions:

1. Whisk all the ingredients in a bowl to make the dough and refrigerate for 10 minutes. Preheat the fryer at 350°F and oil the pan. Pour the dough into the pan, bake for 5 to 7 minutes. Cool and serve the cookies.

27. Jelly Bars

(Ready in about 30 minutes | **Serving:** 8 | **Difficulty**: Easy)

Per serving: **Kcal**: 136, **Fat**: 7 g, **Net Carbs**: 18 g, **Protein**: 3 g

Ingredients:

- ½ cup whole-wheat pastry flour

- ½ teaspoon baking powder

- ¼ teaspoon salt

- 1/3 cup banana, mashed

- ¼ cup smooth natural peanut butter

- 3 tablespoons maple syrup, real

- 2 teaspoons coconut oil, melted

- ½ teaspoon vanilla extract, pure

- 2 tablespoons raw chopped shelled peanuts

- 2 tablespoons raspberry preserves

Instructions:

1. Preheat the fryer at 350°F and oil the pan. Mix peanut butter, maple syrup, coconut oil, and vanilla in one bowl and the rest of the ingredients in another bowl. Add the banana mixture to the flour mixture and pour this batter into the pan. Sprinkle raspberry preserves on the batter as well. Bake this for 20 to 22 minutes. Cool, slice, and serve the bread.

28. Banana & Strawberry Bread

(Ready in about 42 minutes | **Serving:** 10 |

Difficulty: Easy)

Per serving: **Kcal**: 181, **Fat**: 6 g, **Net Carbs**: 30 g,

Protein: 5 g

Ingredients:

- 1 cup + ¼ cup whole-wheat white flour

- 1 cup instant oats

- 1 teaspoon ground cinnamon

- 1 teaspoon + ½ teaspoon baking soda

- 1 cup well-mashed bananas

- 1 egg

- ¼ cup brown sugar, packed and organic

- 2 tablespoon coconut oil, melted

- ¾ cup + 1 tablespoon buttermilk, reduces-fat

- 1 cup strawberries, freeze-dried

- ¼ cup mini semi-sweet chocolate chips

Instructions:

1. Preheat the fryer at 350°F and oil the pan. Mix flour, oats, cinnamon, and baking soda in one bowl and the rest of the ingredients in another bowl. Combine these mixtures and also add strawberries and chocolate chips. Pour this batter into the pan and bake for 23 to 27 minutes. Cool, slice, and serve the bread.

29. Berry Cake

(Ready in about 27 minutes | **Serving:** 1 | **Difficulty:**

Easy)

Per serving: **Kcal**: 269, **Fat**: 15 g, **Net Carbs**: 32 g,

Protein: 4 g

Ingredients:

- 2 tablespoon whole-wheat white flour

- 1 tablespoon+ ½ teaspoon divided brown sugar

- 1/8 teaspoon baking powder

- A pinch of sea salt

- 2 tablespoon milk

- 1/8 teaspoon vanilla extract

- 1 tablespoon grapeseed oil

- 1 teaspoon semi-sweet mini chocolate chips

- ¼ cup berries, frozen

Instructions:

1. Preheat the fryer at 350°F and oil the pan. Mix all the ingredients and make a batter. Pour this batter into the pan and sprinkle it with berries and brown sugar. Bake this for 20 to 24 minutes until brown. Serve.

30. Fruit Tacos

(Ready in about 15 minutes | **Serving:** 4 | **Difficulty**: Easy)

Per serving: **Kcal**: 174, **Fat**: 6 g, **Net Carbs**: 24 g, **Protein**: 7 g

Ingredients:

- Taco dessert shells

- 4 wonton wrappers

- Coconut oil melted

- Cinnamon

- Sugar

- Creamy filling

- 2 tablespoon yogurts

- Citrus peel, grated

- Sweetener: maple syrup, honey, brown sugar

Chopped Fruit:

- Mango, bananas, strawberries, clementine, blackberries, raspberries, apples

Toppings:

- Chocolate chips mini, fresh mint, cooked coconut, chopped nuts

Instructions:

1. Preheat the fryer at 400°F. Put coconut oil on both sides of the wrapper and also drizzle cinnamon and sugar on one side of it. Cover muffin tins with these wrappers and bake for 5 to 7 minutes until crispy. Fill these with the mixture of the rest of the ingredients and serve.

Chapter 6: Pork and Lamb

Recipes

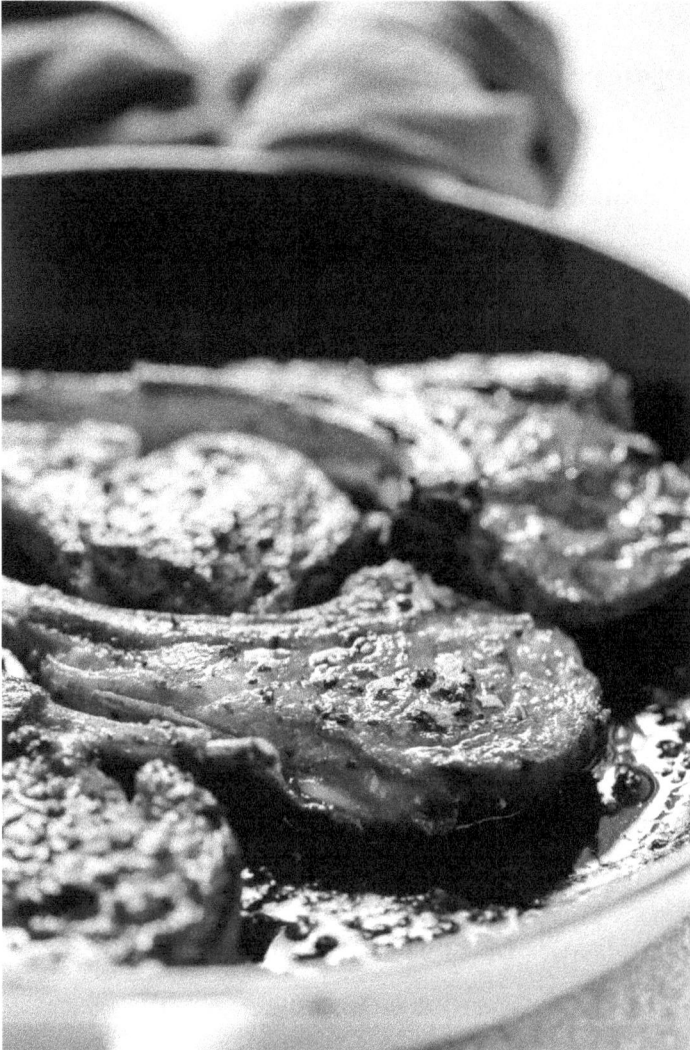

31. Dinner Rolls with Garlic and Tomato Sauce

(Ready in about 20 minutes | **Serving:** 4 | **Difficulty**: Easy)

Per serving: **Kcal:** 217, **Fat**: 5 g, **Net Carbs**: 12 g, **Protein**: 4 g

Ingredients:

- 4 frozen dinner rolls

- 4 minced garlic cloves

- ½ teaspoon dried oregano

- ½ teaspoon garlic powder

- 1 cup of tomato sauce

- Cooking spray

Instructions:

1. Press dinner rolls to form 4 ovals on a working surface. Spray using cooking spray and place them in the basket of the fryer. Toast for around 2 minutes at 370°F. Spread each oval with tomato sauce and divide garlic, sprinkle garlic powder and oregano, and place in the basket again. Toast for around 8 minutes at 370°F.

32. Pork with Potatoes

(Ready in about 35 minutes | **Serving:** 2 | **Difficulty**: Easy)

Per serving: Kcal: 400, **Fat:** 15 g, **Net Carbs**: 27 g, **Protein**: 20 g

Ingredients:

- 2 lbs. pork loin

- Salt

- Black pepper

- 2 sliced as medium wedges red potatoes

- ½ teaspoon garlic powder

- ½ teaspoon pepper flakes

- 1 teaspoon dried parsley

- A drizzle of balsamic vinegar

Instructions:

1. Add all the ingredients to a pan and mix to coat thoroughly. Place in fryer and toast for around 25 minutes at 390°F.

33. Bacon Pudding

(Ready in about 40 minutes | **Serving:** 6 | **Difficulty**:

Easy)

Per serving: **Kcal:** 276, **Fat**: 10 g, **Net Carbs**: 20 g,

Protein: 10 g

Ingredients:

- 4 cooked bacon strips, and chopped

- 1 tablespoon soft butter

- 2 cups corn

- 1 chopped yellow onion

- ¼ cup chopped celery

- ½ cup chopped bell pepper

- 1 teaspoon chopped thyme

- 2 teaspoons minced garlic

- Salt

- Black pepper

- ½ cup of heavy cream

- 1½ cup milk

- 3 whisked eggs

- 3 cups cubed bread

- 4 tablespoons grated parmesan

- Cooking spray

Instructions:

1. Coat pan using cooking spray. Add all the ingredients in a bowl with bacon except cheese and mix to coat evenly. Pour this mixture into

the pan and sprinkle it with cheese. Toast for around 30 minutes at 320°F.

34. Lamb Meatballs

(Ready in about 18 minutes | **Serving:** 10 | **Difficulty**: Easy)

Per serving: **Kcal:** 234, **Fat**: 12 g, **Net Carbs**: 20 g, **Protein**: 30 g

Ingredients:

- 4 oz. minced lamb meat

- Salt

- Black pepper

- 1 toasted bread slice, crumbled

- 2 tablespoon crumbled feta cheese

- ½ tablespoon grated lemon peel

- 1 tablespoon chopped oregano

Instructions:

1. Add all the ingredients with lamb in a bowl and mix thoroughly. Form 10 meatballs out of the mixture and place them in the basket of the fryer. Toast for around 8 minutes at 400°F.

Chapter 7: Poultry Recipes

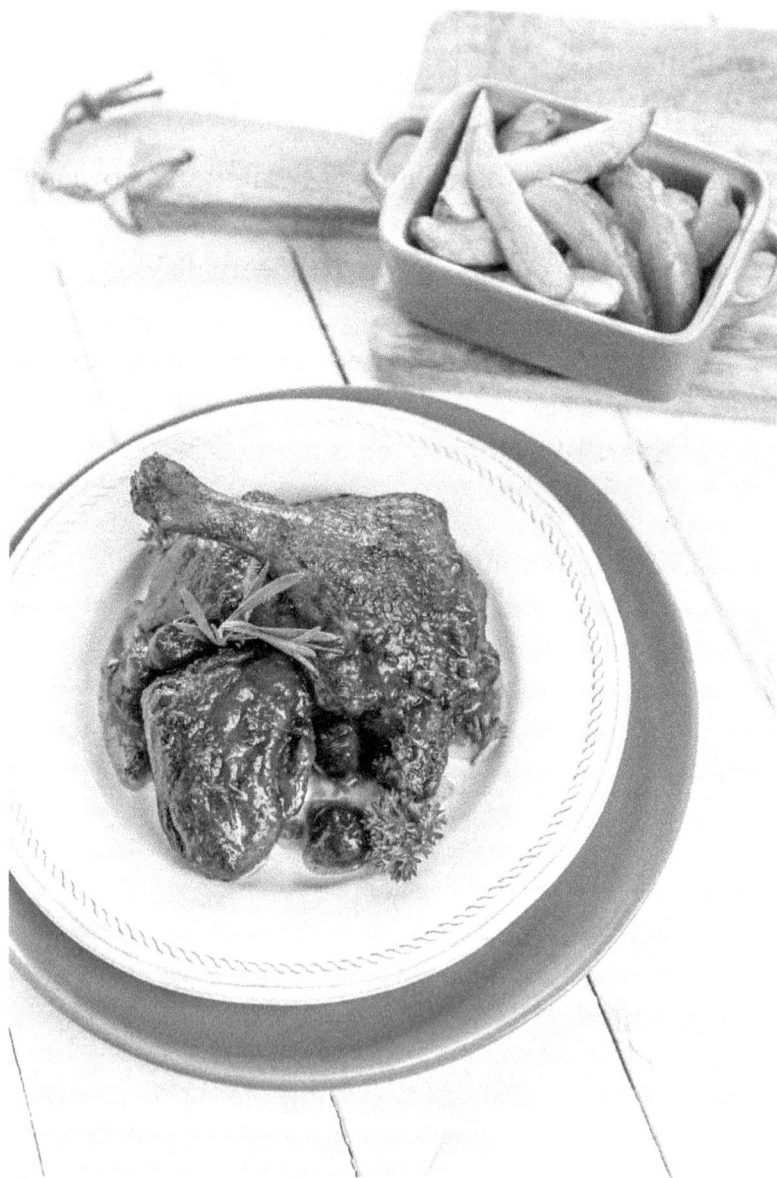

35. Duck with Cherries

(Ready in about 30 minutes | **Serving:** 4 | **Difficulty**: Easy)

Per serving: **Kcal:** 456, **Fat**: 13 g, **Net Carbs**: 64 g, **Protein**: 31 g

Ingredients:

- 1/2 cup sugar

- 1/4 cup honey

- 1/3 cup balsamic vinegar

- 1 teaspoon minced garlic

- 1 tablespoon grated ginger

- 1 teaspoon ground cumin

- 1/2 teaspoon ground clove

- 1/2 teaspoon cinnamon powder

- 4 chopped sage leaves

- 1 chopped jalapeño

- 2 cups sliced rhubarb

- 1/2 cup chopped yellow onion

- 2 cups pitted cherries

- 4 boneless scored duck breasts

- Black pepper and salt

Instructions:

1. Season duck with pepper and salt and place in the basket of the fryer. Broil for around 10 minutes at 350°F. Flip at halftime. Warm a pan and add the rest of the ingredients. Simmer the

mixture and cook for around 10 minutes. Toss

duck in this mixture and enjoy.

36. Marinated Duck

(Ready in about 40 minutes | **Serving:** 4 | **Difficulty**:

Easy)

Per serving: **Kcal:** 475, **Fat:** 12 g, **Net Carbs**: 10 g,

Protein: 48 g

Ingredients:

- 2 duck breasts

- 1 cup white wine

- 1/4 cup soy sauce

- 2 minced garlic cloves

- 6 tarragon sprigs

- Black pepper and salt

- 1 tablespoon butter

- 1/4 cup sherry wine

Instructions:

1. Add duck to bowl with rest of ingredients except sherry and butter. Mix to coat the duck thoroughly and place in the fridge for around one day. Transfer to the basket of the fryer and bake for around 10 minutes at 350°F. Flip at halftime. Add the rest of the ingredients with the marinade in a pan and place on a moderate flame. Cook for around 5 minutes and drizzle sauce over duck.

37. Chicken with Fruit Sauce

(Ready in about 20 minutes | **Serving:** 4 | **Difficulty**: Easy)

Per serving: **Kcal:** 374, **Fat**: 8 g, **Net Carbs**: 34 g, **Protein**: 37 g

Ingredients:

- 4 chicken breasts

- Black pepper and salt

- 4 halved and deseeded passion fruits, pulp reserved

- 1 tablespoon whiskey

- 2 star anise

- 2 oz. maple syrup

- 1 bunch chopped chives

Instructions:

1. Warm a pan with fruit pulp and add star anise, whiskey, chives, and maple syrup. Simmer for around 6 minutes. Season chicken using pepper and salt and place in a basket of fryers. Bake for around 10 minutes at 360°F. Drizzle sauce over chicken and enjoy.

38. Chicken with Radish

(Ready in about 40 minutes | **Serving:** 4 | **Difficulty:** Easy)

Per serving: **Kcal:** 237, **Fat:** 10 g, **Net Carbs**: 19 g, **Protein**: 29 g

Ingredients:

- 4 bone-in chicken thighs

- Black pepper and salt

- 1 tablespoon olive oil

- 1 cup chicken stock

- 6 halved radishes

- 1 teaspoon sugar

- 3 carrots, diced into fine sticks

- 2 tablespoons chopped chives

Instructions:

1. Add stock, sugar, carrots, and radishes in a pan that can be placed inside the fryer and stir. Simmer for around 20 minutes on a moderate flame. Rub chicken with pepper, salt, oil, and

place in the basket of the fryer. Bake for around

4 minutes at 350°F. Add chicken to the mixture

of radish and place in a fryer. Bake for around 4

minutes.

39. Ham with Cauliflower

(Ready in about 1 hour 10 minutes | **Serving:** 6 |

Difficulty: Hard)

Per serving: **Kcal:** 320, **Fat**: 20 g, **Net Carbs**: 16 g,

Protein: 23 g

Ingredients:

- 8 oz. grated cheddar cheese

- 4 cups cubed ham

- 14 oz. chicken stock

- 1/2 teaspoon garlic powder

- 1/2 teaspoon onion powder

- Black pepper and salt

- 4 minced garlic cloves

- 1/4 cup heavy cream

- 16 oz. cauliflower florets

Instructions:

1. Add ham with the rest of the ingredients in a pan that can be placed in your fryer. Toss to combine all the ingredients. Bake for around 60 minutes at 300°F.

40. Crispy Chicken

(Ready in about 30 minutes | **Serving:** 4 | **Difficulty**: Easy)

Per serving: **Kcal**: 651, **Fat**: 18 g, **Net Carbs**: 57 g, **Protein**: 63 g

Ingredients:

- 1 cup quinoa cooked

- 4 skinless, boneless chicken breasts (6 oz. each)

- ¼ cup Dijon mustard

- 1 tablespoon chopped fresh thyme or marjoram

- ½ teaspoon black pepper

- ½ teaspoon kosher salt

- Olive oil spray

Instructions:

1. Preheat the fryer to 300°F. Spread prepared quinoa on a pan and air fry for around 20 minutes. Transfer to a plate and increase the temperature to 375°F. Spray basket using oil and combine rest of ingredients with chicken in a bowl. Coat chicken and dip in quinoa. Place in the basket and air fry for around 20 minutes.

Chapter 8: Vegetable

Recipes

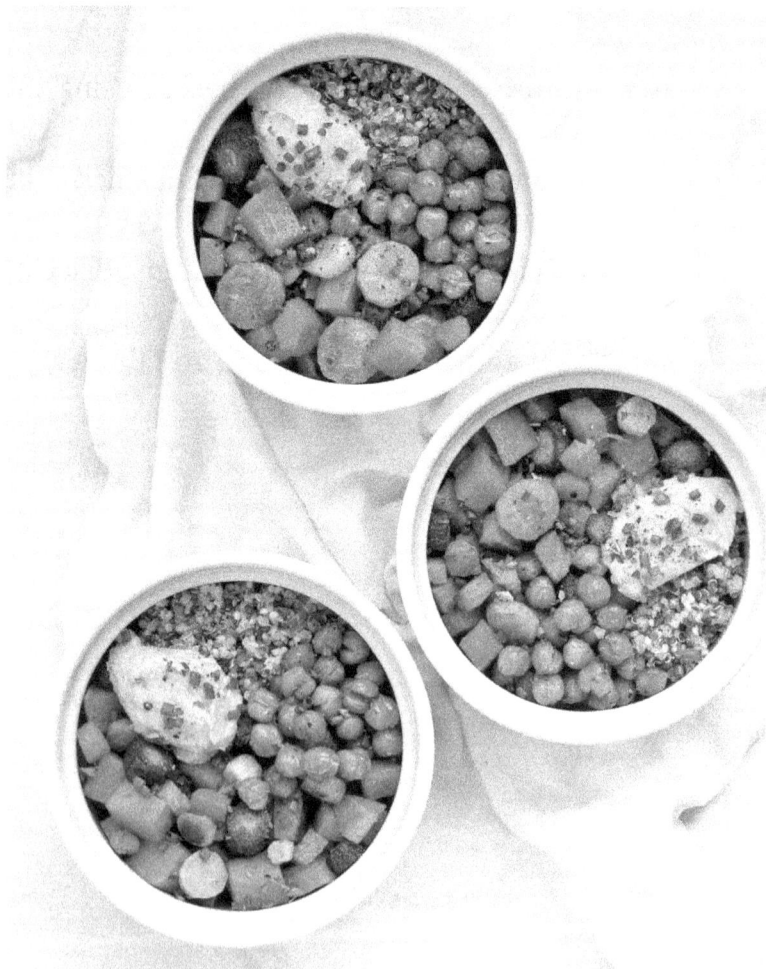

41. Roasted Hummus Bowls

(Ready in about 45 minutes | **Serving:** 2 | **Difficulty**:

Easy)

Per serving: **Kcal:** 469, **Fat**: 22 g, **Net Carbs:** 61 g,

Protein: 17 g

Ingredients:

Roasted Vegetables:

- 10 oz. halved Brussels sprouts

- ½ cup diced yellow bell pepper

- ½ cup red onion, diced

- 4 teaspoons olive oil

- 1 teaspoon any seasoning blend

- Salt

- Pepper

For Bowls:

- 1½–2 cups prepared grains (like brown rice, quinoa, or farro)
- ¼ cup hummus, prepared
- ¼ cup feta cheese, crumbled
- 2 handfuls of baby spinach
- ½ cup sliced grape tomatoes
- 2 teaspoon balsamic vinegar
- 1 lemon, wedged

Instructions:

1. Preheat the fryer to 400°F. Place veggies in a pan and drizzle oil over them. Sprinkle with pepper, seasoning, and salt. Roast for around 30 minutes and flip at half time. Warm grains in microwave and top with hummus, cheese, tomatoes, spinach, and roasted veggies. Drizzle vinegar and enjoy with wedges of lemon.

42. Peanut Butter with Jelly Sandwich

(Ready in about 8 minutes | **Serving:** 1 | **Difficulty**: Easy)

Per serving: **Kcal:** 425, **Fat**: 26 g, **Net Carbs:** 37 g, **Protein**: 14 g

Ingredients:

- 2 bread slices

- 2 teaspoons softened butter

- 2 tablespoons peanut butter

- 1 tablespoon fruit preserves

Instructions:

1. Spread butter on both slices of bread and flip them. Spread peanut butter on this side. Spread one slice with preserves and top with buttered side up of the other bread slice. Place sandwich in pan and toast for around 3 minutes. Allow it to cool before serving.

43. Tacos with Mango

(Ready in about 35 minutes | **Serving:** 4 | **Difficulty**: Easy)

Per serving: **Kcal:** 407, **Fat**: 14 g, **Net Carbs:** 63 g, **Protein**: 11 g

Ingredients:

Roasted Sprouts:

- 8 oz. Brussels sprouts

- 2–3 teaspoon olive oil

- 1 tablespoon taco seasoning

Mango Salsa:

- ½ cup mango, cubed

- ¼ cup roughly chopped cilantro leaves

- 2 tablespoons red onion, chopped

- 1 tablespoon jalapeno, diced

- ½ avocado, cubed

- ½ cup black beans, cooked

- ½ juiced lime

- Salt and pepper, as per taste

For Serving:

- 4 tortillas (corn)

Instructions:

1. Preheat the fryer to 400°F. Dice sprouts and add to bowl. Drizzle them with oil and add taco seasoning. Toss to mix and place in pan in one layer. Toast for around 20 minutes and season with pepper and salt. Add the rest of the ingredients in a bowl in the meantime to form salsa and place in the fridge. Warm tortillas in a pan and fill with salsa and sprouts.

44. Roasted Pita Sandwiches

(Ready in about 30 minutes | **Serving:** 2 | **Difficulty**:

Easy)

Per serving: **Kcal:** 432, **Fat:** 20 g, **Net Carbs:** 53 g,

Protein: 15 g

Ingredients:

- 1 zucchini squash, small

- ½ cup bell pepper, diced

- ½ cup red onion, chopped

- 2 teaspoons olive oil

- ¼ teaspoon dried oregano

- ¼ teaspoon dried thyme

- ¼ teaspoon garlic powder

- Salt

- Pepper

- 2 whole-wheat pitas

- ½ cup hummus

- 1 ½ cups spinach, fresh

- 2 tablespoons feta cheese, crumbled

Instructions:

1. Preheat the fryer to 425°F. Cut the zucchini lengthwise in the quarter and then in pieces of 1/2 inch thickness. Cut onion and bell pepper in pieces of 1-inch thickness. Add veggies to the pan and drizzle with the oil. Sprinkle with seasonings and toss to mix. Toast for around 10 minutes. Stir and toast for another 5 minutes. Warm pitas for around 2 minutes at 375°F and spread them with hummus. Layer spinach, veggies, and feta and enjoy.

45. Cheddar Pizza

(Ready in about 15 minutes | **Serving:** 1 | **Difficulty**:

Easy)

Per serving: **Kcal:** 323, **Fat**: 11 g, **Net Carbs:** 50 g,

Protein: 12 g

Ingredients:

- pita bread

- ½ teaspoon apricot preserves

- 1 tablespoon feta cheese, crumbled

- 2 tablespoons pecans, chopped

- ½ cup loosely packed baby spinach

- ½ thinly sliced apple, seeded

- ½ cup mild cheddar shredded cheese

- Fresh rosemary

Instructions:

1. Preheat the fryer to 400°F. Place pita on the pan and add preserves. Top with half quantity of pecans, feta, and spinach. Add apple slices in a layer of spinach and sprinkle with cheese and the rest of the pecans. Toast for around 11 minutes and top with rosemary.

46. Spaghetti Squash

(Ready in about 1 hour 10 minutes | **Serving:** 2 | **Difficulty**: Hard)

Per serving: **Kcal:** 391, **Fat:** 20 g, **Net Carbs**: 48 g, **Protein**: 10 g

Ingredients:

Spaghetti Squash:

- 30 oz. spaghetti squash

- 1 teaspoon olive oil

- ¼ teaspoon dried oregano

- 1/8 teaspoon garlic powder

- Salt and pepper

Instructions:

1. Preheat the fryer to 425°F and oil a pan. Poke squash with a knife on every side and microwave for around 5 minutes. Slice lengthwise in half and remove seeds. Rub oil and add seasonings. Place squash in pan and toast for around 45

minutes. Scrape to make strands along the flesh.

Divide toppings on squash and enjoy.

47. Jalapeño Grilled Cheese

(Ready in about 25 minutes | **Serving:** 1 | **Difficulty**:

Easy)

Per serving: **Kcal:** 545, **Fat:** 29 g, **Net Carbs:** 51 g,

Protein: 22 g

Ingredients:

- 1 jalapeño

- 2 whole-grain bread slices

- 2 teaspoons mayonnaise

- 1 oz. softened cream cheese

- 1 tablespoon green onions, sliced

- A pinch of garlic powder

- ¼ cup Monterey Jack shredded cheese

- 2 tablespoons mild cheddar shredded cheese

- 2 teaspoons honey

- ¼ cup cereal corn flakes

Instructions:

1. Preheat fryer to 400°F. Slice jalapeno into slices of 1/4 inch and take seeds out. Place on pan and toast for around 4 minutes. Place aside. Spread mayonnaise on each bread slice. Combine the rest of the ingredients except honey and flakes in a bowl. Add this mixture to bread slices and add jalapeno to one slice. Add an equal amount of cheese to bread slices and place in the pan.

Toast for around 7 minutes. Drizzle with honey and flakes and top with the slice.

48. Mushroom Sandwich

(Ready in about 35 minutes | **Serving:** 2 | **Difficulty:** Easy)

Per serving: **Kcal:** 407, **Fat**: 16 g, **Net Carbs**: 52 g, **Protein**: 16 g

Ingredients:

- 2 sandwich rolls
- 2 teaspoons olive oil
- 1 tablespoon balsamic vinegar
- 2 teaspoons soy sauce low sodium
- ½ teaspoon dried oregano

- ¼ teaspoon garlic powder

- ¼ teaspoon black pepper

- 1 large thinly sliced Portobello mushroom

- 1 thinly sliced bell pepper

- ½ thinly sliced small onion

- 2 provolone cheese slices

Instructions:

1. Preheat the fryer to 425°F. Warm sandwich rolls for around one minute. Coat a pan with 1 teaspoon of oil. Add all the ingredients except veggies and cheese to make the sauce. Add veggies to the coat and pour the mixture into the pan. Toast for around 18 minutes and top with

cheese. Toast for 3 more minutes. Split the rolls and fill with mixture and enjoy.

49. Pizza Bagels

(Ready in about 6 hours 21 minutes | **Serving:** 6 | **Difficulty**: Hard)

Per serving: **Kcal:** 160, **Fat**: 3 g, **Net Carbs:** 27 g, **Protein**: 6 g

Ingredients:

- 3 bagels mini

- 6 tablespoon pizza sauce

- ¾ cup mozzarella shredded cheese

- ½–¾ cup toppings (veggies, peppers, and olives)

Instructions:

1. Line a pan with parchment paper. Cut bagel and add to the pan. Top with 2 tablespoons of cheese, 1 tablespoon of pizza sauce, and toppings of choice. Place in freezer for around 8 hours. Preheat the fryer to 400°F. Place pizzas on a pan and toast for around 11 minutes.

50. Caprese Sandwich

(Ready in about 10 minutes | **Serving:** 1 | **Difficulty**:

Easy)

Per serving: **Kcal:** 275354 **Fat**: 16 g, **Net Carbs:** 31

g, **Protein**: 22 g

Ingredients:

- 2 multigrain bread slices

- 2 teaspoons mayonnaise

- 2 mozzarella cheese slices

- 1 fresh tomato (¼" slices)

- 3 fresh thinly sliced basil leaves

- Salt

- Pepper

- A drizzle of balsamic glaze

Instructions:

1. Spread mayonnaise on every slice of bread. Slip and top with a mozzarella slice. Place in the pan with cheese side up and toast for around 5 minutes. Sprinkle basil on both slices equally and add tomato on one. Season with pepper and salt and drizzle glaze. Place the other piece on top and enjoy.

Conclusion

Air fryers function mostly by the circulation of hot air around the food dish, which gradually cooks it. The air that comes out of the fans cooks the food in a way similar to oil fryers, leaving the exterior very crispy due to the electric power. In short, frying food in a hot air fryer is a much healthier way of eating it.

In fact, as opposed to conventional oil fryers, cooking food in a hot air fryer is a much better form of eating it. In addition to being much better, so we stop consuming so much fat, hot air fryers will cook a wide range of meals; there are no limitations to the variety of balanced recipes that anyone can enjoy.

Your imagination is the limit when it comes to creating these delicious dishes or complementing a meal with a crunchier touch. The important thing is to know how to combine various ingredients that will give that special touch to your dishes and highlight your culinary skills.

CPSIA information can be obtained
at www.ICGtesting.com
Printed in the USA
BVHW040257080521
606756BV00005B/1301

9 781801 566483